Enlightened Rest - 20 Transformative Yoga Nidra Practices for Spiritual and Yoga Teachers
By Ristha Sanei

Contents

Connection with Earth: Foster a sense of grounding by guiding participants to connect with the Earth's energy and draw strength from it.	31
Candle Flame Concentration: Use the image of a candle flame to enhance concentration and focus, allowing the mind to settle.	33
Muscle Relaxation Journey: Lead a journey where participants systematically relax and release tension from each muscle group.	35
Mindful Eating Experience: Incorporate mindfulness into the practice by guiding participants through a visualization of a mindful eating experience.	37
Dream Exploration: Encourage participants to explore the realm of dreams, unlocking insights and creativity within their subconscious mind.	39
Colourful Energy Flow: Guide participants to visualize and feel the flow of colorful, positive energy throughout their body.	41
Breathing with the Elements: Connect breathwork with the elements (earth, air, water, fire), creating a harmonious experience with nature.	44

Introduction

What is a Yoga Nidra?

Yoga Nidra, often referred to as yogic sleep, is a systematic and guided relaxation practice that leads participants into a state of conscious relaxation between wakefulness and sleep. The term "Yoga Nidra" is derived from two Sanskrit words: "yoga," meaning union or integration, and "nidra," meaning sleep. Despite the name, the aim is not to fall asleep but to reach a state of deep relaxation while maintaining a trace of awareness.

In a typical Yoga Nidra session, participants lie down in a comfortable and supported position, often in Savasana (corpse pose). The facilitator then guides them through a series of instructions and visualize actions to promote relaxation at physical, mental, and emotional levels.

Key elements of a Yoga Nidra session may include:

1. **Body Scan:** Participants bring their awareness to different parts of the body, systematically releasing tension and promoting a sense of relaxation.
2. **Breath Awareness:** Focusing on the natural breath, participants observe the inhalation and exhalation, bringing attention to the rhythm and sensations of breathing.
3. **Visualizations:** Guided imagery is used to create a mental landscape, allowing participants to explore various scenes, symbols, or experiences that promote relaxation and well-being.
4. **Intention Setting:** Participants may be encouraged to set a positive intention or Sankalpa for the practice, aligning with their deeper desires and goals.
5. **Body Rotation:** Moving attention through different parts of the body, participants deepen their relaxation and cultivate a sense of stillness.
6. **Awareness of Sensations and Emotions:** Participants may be guided to observe and accept sensations, emotions, and thoughts without attachment or judgment.
7. **Time Distortion:** The perception of time may be altered, with a few minutes in reality feeling like a longer period during the practice.

The ultimate goal of Yoga Nidra is to induce a state of profound relaxation, allowing for physical and mental healing, stress reduction, and enhanced self-awareness. It is often used as a tool for managing stress, anxiety, insomnia, and promoting overall well-being. A typical session can range from 20 minutes to an hour, depending on the specific goals and context.

There are 20 Yoga Nidra that you can use during Savasana (Corpse Pose)

1. Mountain Visualization

Welcome, everyone. Find a cozy spot, lie down, and let's embark on a journey of relaxation. Close your eyes and take a deep breath, releasing any tension or worries. Feel your body sinking into the surface beneath you as you let go.

Now, shift your focus to your toes. Imagine warm, golden sunlight gently caressing your toes, melting away any tightness. Picture the sensation of soft, cool grass beneath your feet, grounding you to the Earth. Move your awareness upward, allowing this soothing energy to flow through each part of your body, like a gentle stream.

As you continue to breathe, imagine the air you inhale is pure, crisp mountain air. As you exhale, visualize releasing any remaining tension, watching it dissipate into the atmosphere. Feel a light breeze brushing against your skin, carrying away any worries or stress.

Now, let's enter the world of the mountain. Visualize yourself on the slope of a grand mountain, surrounded by vibrant wildflowers. As you ascend, notice the textures of the earth beneath your feet – smooth rocks, soft moss, and the occasional crunch of fallen leaves.

Gaze at the panoramic view from the mountain's peak. Below, see a serene valley with a meandering river reflecting the colors of the setting sun. Above, the sky transforms into a canvas of warm hues, casting a golden glow over everything.

You are the mountain – solid, majestic, and unyielding. Sense the strength of the mountain within you, and feel the stability grounding you deep into the Earth. Visualize the mountain's summit reaching into the vast sky, connecting with the infinite.

Embrace a moment of silence here, absorbing the serenity of this mountain landscape.

[Pause]

As you gently return to awareness, feel the warmth of the sun on your skin. Picture yourself slowly descending the mountain, leaving behind any tension or worries with each step. The air becomes lighter, and you feel a renewed sense of energy.

Begin to deepen your breath, allowing the crisp mountain air to invigorate your entire being. As you open your eyes, carry the strength and tranquility of the mountain with you into the rest of your day.

Thank you for joining me in this Mountain Visualization. Take a moment to express gratitude for the time you spent in this rejuvenating journey. When you're ready, gently open your eyes and return to the present moment

2.
Ocean Waves Relaxation

"Welcome, everyone. Let's find a comfortable position lying down. Close your eyes and take a moment to settle into stillness. Inhale deeply, and as you exhale, let go of any tension or thoughts that may be lingering from your day. Feel the support beneath you and allow your body to surrender to the ground.

[Pause]

As you settle in, become aware of your breath. Inhale and exhale naturally, feeling the gentle rise and fall of your chest. Imagine that with each breath, you are drawing in the calm energy of the ocean.

Now, visualize yourself on a peaceful beach. Picture the golden sand beneath you, soft and warm. Feel the gentle caress of the ocean breeze on your skin. As you continue to breathe, hear the rhythmic sound of waves breaking on the shore, creating a soothing melody.

[Pause]

As we begin our journey, let's bring our attention to the toes. Imagine the waves gently washing over your toes, releasing any tension. Feel the cool, refreshing sensation as the waves recede.

Now, the waves move up to your ankles, and you sense a gentle, swirling current around your feet. Let go of any heaviness or discomfort, allowing the waves to carry it away.

[Pause]

The waves continue their journey, reaching your knees. Feel a sense of relaxation and release as the water massages and cleanses each leg.

[Pause]

Now, the waves embrace your hips, allowing you to surrender into their calming rhythm. Sense any tightness or tension dissolving with each wave that washes over you.

[Pause]

The ocean waves now move up to your chest and shoulders. As they flow over you, let go of any burdens or stress you may be carrying. Feel a sense of weightlessness and ease.

[Pause]

Sense the waves gently moving down your arms, from the shoulders to the fingertips. Your arms become weightless, carried by the gentle ebb and flow of the ocean.

[Pause]

Now, the waves reach your neck and head. Feel the soothing water enveloping you, allowing your neck to relax, and your head to be cradled by the gentle movements of the ocean.

[Pause]

You are now completely immersed in the ocean of relaxation. Imagine floating effortlessly, supported by the vastness of the sea. Take a moment to enjoy this sensation, surrendering to the tranquil energy around you.

[Pause]

As we gradually conclude our practice, become aware of your breath once again. Feel the ocean waves slowly receding, leaving you with a profound sense of peace and serenity.

[Pause]

Start to bring awareness back to your surroundings. Begin to gently wiggle your fingers and toes, inviting movement back into your body. When you're ready, slowly and mindfully, open your eyes.

Thank you for joining me in this Ocean Waves Relaxation. Carry this sense of calm and tranquility with you as you continue with your day. Namaste."

3. Forest Retreat Yoga Nidra

Welcome, dear friends. Let's begin our journey into deep relaxation. Find a comfortable position lying down, close your eyes, and take a few moments to settle into the stillness. Inhale deeply, and as you exhale, release any tension or worries you may be carrying. Feel the support beneath you, allowing your body to melt into the ground.

[Pause]

Imagine yourself standing at the edge of a lush and tranquil forest. Picture the towering trees surrounding you, their branches reaching up to the sky. The air is filled with the earthy scent of moss, and a gentle breeze rustles the leaves overhead.

As you stand there, become aware of your breath. Inhale the fresh forest air, and with each exhale, let go of any lingering thoughts. Sense the connection between your breath and the rhythm of the forest.

[Pause]

Now, let's take a mindful journey through the forest.

Begin by feeling the soft forest floor beneath your feet. Picture the ground covered in a thick layer of moss, providing a cushion for each step you take. As you walk, notice the coolness and support of the moss beneath you.

[Pause]

Moving deeper into the forest, you encounter a babbling brook. Imagine the soothing sound of the water flowing over smooth stones. Allow the sound to wash over you, calming your mind and inviting a sense of serenity.

[Pause]

Continuing your journey, you come across a peaceful clearing bathed in dappled sunlight. Feel the warmth on your skin as you step into the clearing. In the center, there's a comfortable spot to rest. As you settle in, you realize you are surrounded by gentle woodland creatures, creating a harmonious atmosphere.

[Pause]

Now, let's bring awareness to different parts of your body. Visualize the trees overhead extending their branches down to gently touch your fingertips, offering a sense of connection and support.

[Pause]

Feel the energy of the forest enveloping you, nurturing and revitalizing every cell of your body. Imagine the trees acting as conduits for grounding energy, allowing you to release any tension or heaviness.

[Pause]

As we conclude our time in the forest, take a moment to express gratitude for the healing energy it provided. Feel a deep sense of relaxation as you prepare to return to your daily life.

[Pause]

Start to bring awareness back to your breath. Begin to gently move your fingers and toes, reconnecting with your physical body. When you're ready, open your eyes, bringing the tranquility of the forest retreat with you.

Thank you for joining me in this Forest Retreat. May the peace and strength of the forest accompany you as you move through your day. Namaste.

4.Body Scan for Relaxation

Welcome, everyone. Find a comfortable position lying down, close your eyes, and take a moment to settle into stillness. Allow your body to rest fully on the ground, releasing any tension from your muscles. Take a deep breath in, and as you exhale, let go of the busyness of your day.

[Pause]

Now, bring your awareness to your toes. Feel the sensation in each toe, as if they are gently sighing and relaxing. Let the soothing wave of relaxation move through your feet, allowing the muscles to soften and release.

[Pause]

Now, shift your attention to your ankles. Imagine a warm, comforting light gently surrounding and loosening any tightness in this area. Feel the tension melting away with each breath.

[Pause]

Move your awareness up to your calves. Picture a soft, golden light bathing your calves, bringing a sense of tranquility. Allow this light to dissolve any tension or fatigue stored in the muscles.

[Pause]

Bring your attention to your knees. Feel a gentle breeze passing over your knees, soothing and calming. Let any discomfort or tightness be carried away with the breeze.

[Pause]

Now, focus on your thighs. Imagine a warm, relaxing energy flowing through your thighs, easing any remaining tension. Sense the muscles becoming soft and pliant.

[Pause]

Shift your awareness to your hips and pelvis. Feel a sense of groundedness and stability in this area. Allow any stress or tension to melt away, leaving you with a feeling of support.

[Pause]

Move up to your lower back. Picture a gentle massage, easing any knots or tightness along your spine. Feel the vertebrae gently aligning, creating space and comfort.

[Pause]

Now, bring your attention to your abdomen. Imagine a warm, golden light embracing your abdomen, promoting relaxation and a sense of ease. Let any holding in this area soften.

[Pause]

Shift your focus to your chest. Feel the rise and fall of your chest with each breath, a natural and soothing rhythm. Sense your heart space opening to a feeling of calmness.

[Pause]

Move to your fingertips. Imagine a soft, warm energy flowing through each fingertip, releasing any tension. Feel a gentle tingling sensation as your fingers relax completely.

[Pause]

Now, bring your attention to your hands and wrists. Picture a stream of cool water washing away any stress, leaving your hands light and free.

[Pause]

Move up to your forearms. Sense a wave of relaxation moving through your forearms, allowing the muscles to loosen and let go.

[Pause]

Now, focus on your elbows. Feel any tightness or resistance in this area dissolving with each breath, creating space for relaxation.

[Pause]

Shift your awareness to your upper arms. Imagine a gentle breeze passing over your upper arms, carrying away any lingering tension. Allow the muscles to soften and release.

[Pause]

Bring your attention to your shoulders. Feel a sense of weight lifting off your shoulders as they relax and settle. Let go of any burdens you may be carrying.

[Pause]

Now, move to your neck. Picture a soft, warm light enveloping your neck, releasing any tightness. Allow your head to feel weightless, supported by the ground beneath.

[Pause]

Shift your focus to your jaw. Allow your jaw to unclench, letting the muscles relax. Feel the space between your teeth, and let go of any tension in your facial muscles.

[Pause]

Now, bring your awareness to your face. Imagine a gentle touch, smoothing away any furrows or lines. Feel the entire face relaxing, and let the forehead become smooth and calm.

[Pause]

Finally, focus on the crown of your head. Picture a soft, golden light gently cradling the crown, creating a sense of openness and tranquility.

[Pause]

Take a moment to scan your entire body. Feel the deep sense of relaxation and peace that has settled within. Your entire being is now in a state of calm and stillness.

[Pause]

As we conclude our Body Scan for Relaxation, slowly begin to bring awareness back to your breath. Gently wiggle your fingers and toes, allowing a sense of awakening to return.

[Pause]

When you feel ready, slowly and mindfully, open your eyes.

Thank you for joining me in this Body Scan for Relaxation. May the serenity and calmness you've cultivated stay with you as you continue your day. Namaste.

5. Gratitude Journey

Welcome, dear practitioners. Let's embark on a journey of deep relaxation and gratitude. Find a comfortable position lying down, close your eyes, and take a moment to settle into the present moment. Inhale deeply, and as you exhale, release any tension or worries that may be lingering from your day.

[Pause]

Now, let's bring our awareness to the breath. Inhale the nourishing air, and with each exhale, let go of any thoughts that may distract you. Allow your breath to guide you into a state of calm and presence.

[Pause]

Imagine yourself in a serene meadow surrounded by nature's beauty. Picture the vibrant colors of flowers, the gentle rustling of leaves, and the clear, open sky above. Feel the soft grass beneath you as you lie down, supported by the Earth.

[Pause]

In this moment, bring to mind something you are truly grateful for. It could be a person, a place, an experience, or even a quality within yourself. Feel the warmth of gratitude expanding in your heart as you focus on this precious aspect of your life.

[Pause]

Now, let that feeling of gratitude extend outward, like rays of sunlight reaching out from your heart. Picture these rays touching the elements around you, infusing the meadow with a radiant, positive energy.

[Pause]

As we continue our journey, let's express gratitude for the physical body that supports us. Bring awareness to your toes, appreciating the simple gift of mobility and sensation in your feet. Feel gratitude for the ability to stand and walk, allowing your toes to relax.

[Pause]

Move your attention to your ankles. Express gratitude for the stability and flexibility they provide. Picture a gentle, soothing light enveloping your ankles, releasing any tension.

[Pause]

Now, focus on your calves. Feel gratitude for the strength that allows you to move and explore the world. Picture a warm, golden light bathing your calves, bringing relaxation and ease.

[Pause]

Shift your awareness to your knees. Express gratitude for the ability to bend and move freely. Picture a soft breeze passing over your knees, soothing and calming any discomfort.

[Pause]

Move up to your thighs. Feel gratitude for the power and support they offer. Imagine a vibrant, healing energy flowing through your thighs, releasing any remaining tension.

[Pause]

Express gratitude for the pelvis and hips, the foundation of your physical body. Picture a sense of stability and balance as you feel a warm, grounding energy in this area.

[Pause]

Now, bring your attention to the abdomen. Feel gratitude for the intricate workings of your digestive system. Imagine a soft, golden light embracing your abdomen, promoting relaxation and well-being.

[Pause]

Shift your focus to the chest. Express gratitude for the heart, the center of love and compassion. Feel a sense of openness and warmth in your chest, as if the heart is expanding with gratitude.

[Pause]

Move to your fingertips. Express gratitude for the dexterity and touch they provide. Picture a gentle stream of cool water washing away any stress, leaving your fingers light and free.

[Pause]

Now, bring your awareness to your hands and wrists. Express gratitude for the ability to create, touch, and connect with the world around you. Feel a soft, warm energy flowing through each hand, bringing relaxation.

[Pause]

Move up to your forearms. Express gratitude for the strength and flexibility they offer. Sense a wave of relaxation moving through your forearms, allowing the muscles to loosen.

[Pause]

Now, focus on your elbows. Express gratitude for the range of motion they provide. Picture a gentle breeze passing over your elbows, carrying away any tension.

[Pause]

Shift your awareness to your upper arms. Express gratitude for the power and strength they offer. Imagine a gentle breeze passing over your upper arms, bringing a sense of lightness.

[Pause]

Bring your attention to your shoulders. Express gratitude for the burdens they carry and the strength they provide. Feel any tension lifting off your shoulders as they relax and settle.

[Pause]

Now, move to your neck. Express gratitude for the ability to turn and nod, connecting with the world around you. Picture a soft, warm light enveloping your neck, releasing any tightness.

[Pause]

Focus on your jaw. Express gratitude for the ability to speak and taste the flavors of life. Allow your jaw to unclench, letting the muscles relax. Feel the space between your teeth.

[Pause]

Move to your face. Express gratitude for the senses – sight, hearing, taste, and smell. Imagine a gentle touch, smoothing away any furrows or lines. Feel the entire face relaxing, and let the forehead become smooth and calm.

[Pause]

Now, bring your awareness to the crown of your head. Express gratitude for the thoughts and ideas that flow through your mind. Picture a soft, golden light gently cradling the crown, creating a sense of openness and tranquility.

[Pause]

As we conclude our Gratitude Journey, take a moment to feel the deep sense of appreciation and thankfulness within your heart. Allow this feeling to radiate throughout your entire being.

[Pause]

Slowly begin to bring awareness back to your breath. Gently wiggle your fingers and toes, allowing a sense of awakening to return.

[Pause]

When you feel ready, slowly and mindfully, open your eyes.

Thank you for joining me in this Gratitude Journey. May the warmth of gratitude stay with you as you continue your day. Namaste."

6. Chakra Balancing

Welcome, dear practitioners. Today, we embark on a journey of chakra balancing to harmonize and align the energy centers within. Find a comfortable position lying down, close your eyes, and take a moment to let go of the outside world. Inhale deeply, and as you exhale, release any tension or worries that may be lingering.

[Pause]

Let's begin by bringing our awareness to the base of the spine, the Muladhara Chakra. Visualize a vibrant, red energy glowing at the base of your spine. This is your foundation, your connection to the Earth. Feel the warmth and stability of this red light as it grounds you securely.

[Pause]

Now, shift your attention to the area just below the navel, the Svadhisthana Chakra. Picture a warm, orange light emanating from this space. Feel the creative and sensual energy flowing, allowing a sense of joy and emotional well-being to blossom.

[Pause]

Move up to the solar plexus, the Manipura Chakra, located in the upper abdomen. Imagine a radiant, yellow light shining brightly. Feel the power and confidence of this yellow light, igniting your inner strength and courage.

[Pause]

Next, bring your focus to the heart center, the Anahata Chakra. Visualize a beautiful, green light expanding from your chest. Feel the gentle warmth and compassion radiating from this green light, connecting you to love and harmony.

[Pause]

Now, shift your awareness to the throat, the Vishuddha Chakra. Picture a soothing, blue light glowing in the throat area. Feel the calm and clear communication that emanates from this blue light, allowing your authentic voice to be heard.

[Pause]

Move up to the space between the eyebrows, the Ajna Chakra. Visualize an indigo light shining brightly. Feel the intuition and inner wisdom that comes from this indigo light, guiding you on your path with clarity.

[Pause]

Finally, bring your attention to the crown of your head, the Sahasrara Chakra. Imagine a radiant, violet light expanding from the crown. Feel a sense of connection to the divine and the vast universe, as this violet light opens you to higher states of consciousness.

[Pause]

Now, as we continue our Chakra Balancing, visualize a column of white light flowing from the base of your spine to the crown of your head. Picture this light gently spiraling and cleansing each chakra, harmonizing the energy flow within.

[Pause]

Feel the entire body immersed in this white light, as it continues to move through you, aligning and balancing each energy center. Sense a profound state of inner harmony and balance as the white light infuses every cell of your being.

[Pause]

As we conclude our Chakra Balancing journey, take a moment to express gratitude for the balance and alignment you've cultivated within. Feel a deep sense of connection to your inner self and the energy that surrounds you.

[Pause]

Slowly begin to bring awareness back to your breath. Gently wiggle your fingers and toes, allowing a sense of awakening to return.

[Pause]

When you feel ready, slowly and mindfully, open your eyes.

Thank you for joining me in this Chakra Balancing practice. May the harmonious energy you've cultivated guide you on your journey. Namaste."

7. Healing Light Meditation

Welcome, dear practitioners. Today, we embark on a Healing Light Meditation journey to nourish and revitalize your entire being. Find a comfortable position lying down, close your eyes, and take a moment to transition into a state of deep relaxation. Inhale deeply, and as you exhale, release any tension or concerns that may be lingering.

[Pause]

As we begin, imagine a gentle, warm light hovering just above the crown of your head. This is the healing light – a radiant, golden energy that holds the power to rejuvenate and restore.

[Pause]

Allow this healing light to descend slowly, like a soft mist, enveloping the crown of your head. Feel its warmth as it permeates your scalp, soothing any tension or stress that may be stored there.

[Pause]

Sense the healing light flowing down to your forehead, releasing any furrows or lines. Feel a sense of calm washing over you as this golden energy moves down to your eyes, your cheeks, and your jaw.

[Pause]

Let the healing light gently touch your neck and throat, creating space and relaxation in these areas. Feel any tightness or constriction dissolve as the light continues its descent.

[Pause]

Now, allow the healing light to move into your shoulders. Sense the warmth spreading across your shoulders, melting away any burdens you may carry. Feel a lightness and ease settling in.

[Pause]

As the healing light progresses, let it flow down your arms, from your upper arms to your elbows and down to your fingertips. Picture the light infusing every cell, bringing a revitalizing energy to your entire being.

[Pause]

Feel the warmth as the healing light moves into your chest, illuminating your heart center. Sense a profound feeling of love and compassion spreading through your chest, healing and nourishing your heart space.

[Pause]

Continue to let the healing light descend, moving through your abdomen and lower back. Feel any tension dissolving as this golden energy works its magic, restoring balance and vitality.

[Pause]

Now, visualize the healing light reaching your hips, thighs, and knees. Sense the soothing warmth as it permeates these areas, releasing any tightness and promoting a deep sense of relaxation.

[Pause]

Allow the healing light to flow down your calves and ankles, moving towards your feet. Picture this golden energy grounding you, connecting you to the Earth's healing energy.

[Pause]

Now, your entire body is bathed in the healing light – a luminous, golden glow that emanates from every pore. Feel a sense of wholeness, balance, and well-being.

[Pause]

As we conclude our Healing Light Meditation, take a moment to bask in the radiant energy surrounding you. Express gratitude for the healing you've allowed into your body, mind, and spirit.

[Pause]

Extend your awareness beyond your physical form. Picture the healing light expanding outward, creating a cocoon of positive energy around you. Feel this cocoon of light as a protective and nourishing force that stays with you throughout your day.

[Pause]

Slowly begin to bring awareness back to your breath. Gently wiggle your fingers and toes, allowing a sense of awakening to return.

[Pause]

When you feel ready, slowly and mindfully, open your eyes.

Thank you for joining me in this Healing Light Meditation. May the radiant energy you've cultivated guide you on your journey to well-being. Namaste.

8. Inner Sanctuary Exploration

"Welcome, dear practitioners. Today, we embark on a journey of Inner Sanctuary Exploration, a tranquil odyssey into the depths of your being. Find a comfortable position lying down, close your eyes, and take a moment to release the external world. Inhale deeply, and as you exhale, let go of any tension or concerns that may linger.

[Pause]

As we begin, picture yourself standing at the entrance of a serene forest. Feel the cool, inviting breeze and the soft earth beneath your feet. Ahead lies a path leading you deeper into the heart of this magical sanctuary.

[Pause]

With each step, sense the weight of the world lifting off your shoulders. As you venture further into the forest, notice the dappled sunlight filtering through the leaves, casting a gentle glow on your path.

[Pause]

Ahead, you discover a clearing, bathed in a soft, golden light. In the center of this clearing stands a majestic tree, its branches reaching skyward. Approach this tree and feel a profound sense of peace emanating from its ancient presence.

[Pause]

As you stand beneath the tree, notice a door carved into its trunk. Open the door and step into a space of pure tranquility. You find yourself in a serene inner sanctuary, a place that is uniquely yours.

[Pause]

Take a moment to explore this sanctuary. Notice the colors, textures, and sounds around you. Perhaps there's a comfortable resting spot or a body of water that reflects the tranquility within.

[Pause]

In this sanctuary, you are completely safe and at peace. Allow any tension or worries to melt away as you immerse yourself in the soothing energy of this inner haven.

[Pause]

Now, bring your attention to your breath. Inhale the pure, rejuvenating air of your sanctuary, and as you exhale, release any remaining tension. Feel a deep sense of calm settling within you.

[Pause]

In this sacred space, you have the power to cultivate positive intentions. What aspect of your being would you like to nurture and strengthen today? Is it patience, gratitude, or self-love? Choose one quality, and let it fill your entire being.

[Pause]

As you bask in the nurturing energy of your inner sanctuary, let this chosen quality permeate every cell of your being. Feel it growing stronger with each breath, anchoring itself into your heart.

[Pause]

Now, express gratitude for the sanctuary within you. Know that you can return to this space whenever you need a moment of calm and self-reflection.

[Pause]

As we gradually conclude our Inner Sanctuary Exploration, take a moment to sense the tranquility that now resides within you. Slowly become aware of your physical body and the environment around you.

[Pause]

When you feel ready, gently begin to bring movement back into your fingers and toes. Take a few deep breaths, and when you're ready, open your eyes.

Thank you for joining me in this Inner Sanctuary Exploration. May the peace you've discovered within guide you on your journey. Namaste."

9. Breath Awareness

Welcome, dear friends. Let's embark on a journey of deep relaxation through breath awareness. Find a comfortable position lying down, close your eyes, and take a few moments to settle into the stillness. Inhale deeply, and as you exhale, release any tension or worries you may be carrying. Feel the support beneath you, allowing your body to melt into the ground.

[Pause]

Now, shift your focus to your breath. Notice the natural rhythm of your inhalations and exhalations. Feel the coolness of the air as you breathe in, and the warmth as you breathe out. Let your breath be your guide as you sink deeper into relaxation.

[Pause]

Imagine each breath as a gentle wave washing over you, cleansing you of any stress or tension. With each inhale, feel yourself expanding and filling with peace. With each exhale, feel yourself surrendering more deeply into relaxation.

[Pause]

As you continue to breathe mindfully, imagine a soft breeze moving through your body, carrying away any remaining worries or distractions. Sense the connection between your breath and the rhythm of the universe, syncing your energy with the flow of life.

[Pause]

Now, let's deepen our awareness of the breath. With each inhale, visualize your lungs filling with bright, healing light, energizing every cell of your body. With each exhale, imagine releasing any stagnant energy or negativity, allowing it to dissolve into the space around you.

[Pause]

As you immerse yourself in the rhythm of your breath, feel a sense of calmness and clarity washing over you. Let go of any thoughts or judgments, and simply be present with your breath.

[Pause]

Know that in this moment, you are fully supported by the nourishing power of your breath. Allow yourself to rest in this awareness, feeling grounded and centered in the present moment.

[Pause]

As we continue to deepen our breath awareness practice, let's explore the sensation of the breath as it moves through different parts of the body. With each inhale, feel the expansion of your belly as it fills with air. With each exhale, feel the gentle release of tension from your shoulders and jaw.

[Pause]

Now, bring your awareness to the rise and fall of your chest with each breath. Notice how your ribs expand and contract with each inhale and exhale, like the gentle movement of ocean waves.

[Pause]

As you continue to breathe deeply, imagine a warm, golden light surrounding you, radiating from the center of your being. With each breath, allow this light to expand, filling the space around you with warmth and love.

[Pause]

Feel the energy of this light infusing every cell of your body, revitalizing and rejuvenating you from within. Let go of any remaining resistance or tension, and surrender to the healing power of your breath.

[Pause]

Know that in this sacred space of breath awareness, you are free to let go of the past and future, and simply be present in the here and now. Allow yourself to rest in this state of deep relaxation for a few moments longer.

[Pause]

As we conclude our breath awareness practice, take a moment to express gratitude for the healing energy it provided. Feel a deep sense of relaxation as you prepare to return to your daily life.

[Pause]

Start to bring awareness back to your physical body. Gently wiggle your fingers and toes, and when you're ready, slowly open your eyes, carrying the tranquility of your breath awareness practice with you.

Thank you for joining me in this extended Breath Awareness Yoga Nidra. May the peace and strength of your breath accompany you as you move through your day. Namaste.

10. **Loving-Kindness Meditation**

Welcome, dear friends. Today, we embark on a journey of loving-kindness meditation. Find a comfortable position lying down, close your eyes, and take a few moments to settle into the stillness. Inhale deeply, and as you exhale, release any tension or worries you may be carrying. Feel the support beneath you, allowing your body to melt into the ground.

[Pause]

Now, bring your attention to your heart center, the seat of compassion and love. Take a moment to connect with your own heart, feeling its warmth and presence within you. Visualize a soft, glowing light radiating from your heart, filling the space around you with love and compassion.

[Pause]

As you sit in this space of loving-kindness, think of someone in your life who fills your heart with love and joy. It could be a friend, a family member, or even a pet. Picture their smiling face before you, radiating with happiness and kindness.

[Pause]

With each inhale, imagine drawing in this love and joy from the person you are visualizing, allowing it to fill your heart to the brim. With each exhale, send this love back out to them, surrounding them with warmth and compassion.

[Pause]

Now, extend this loving-kindness to yourself. Visualize your own reflection in a mirror, looking at yourself with eyes of love and acceptance. Repeat the following phrases silently to yourself, allowing the words to resonate deeply within you: "May I be happy. May I be healthy. May I be safe. May I be at peace."

[Pause]

Feel the loving-kindness flowing freely from your heart, enveloping both yourself and others in its gentle embrace. Allow yourself to bask in this warm, loving energy for a few moments, knowing that you are deserving of love and compassion, just as much as anyone else.

[Pause]

Now, expand your circle of loving-kindness to include all beings, near and far, known and unknown. Visualize the entire world bathed in this radiant light of love and compassion, bringing healing and peace to all.

[Pause]

As we conclude our loving-kindness meditation, take a moment to express gratitude for the love and connection you've cultivated. Feel a deep sense of peace and warmth as you prepare to return to your daily life.

[Pause]

Start to bring awareness back to your physical body. Gently wiggle your fingers and toes, and when you're ready, slowly open your eyes, carrying the love and compassion of this meditation with you.

Thank you for joining me in this Loving-Kindness Meditation Yoga Nidra. May the love and kindness you've cultivated here ripple out into the world, touching the hearts of all beings. May you carry this warmth and compassion with you as you navigate your journey ahead. Namaste.

11.Stress Release through Symbolism

Welcome, dear friends. Today, we embark on a journey of stress release through symbolism. Find a comfortable position lying down, close your eyes, and take a few moments to settle into the stillness. Inhale deeply, and as you exhale, release any tension or worries you may be carrying. Feel the support beneath you, allowing your body to melt into the ground.

[Pause]

Imagine yourself standing at the edge of a lush and tranquil forest. Picture the towering trees surrounding you, their branches reaching up to the sky. The air is filled with the earthy scent of moss, and a gentle breeze rustles the leaves overhead.

[Pause]

As you stand there, become aware of your breath. Inhale the fresh forest air, and with each exhale, let go of any lingering thoughts. Sense the connection between your breath and the rhythm of the forest.

[Pause]

Now, let's take a mindful journey through the forest. Begin by feeling the soft forest floor beneath your feet. Picture the ground covered in a thick layer of moss, providing a cushion for each step you take. As you walk, notice the coolness and support of the moss beneath you.

[Pause]

Moving deeper into the forest, you encounter a babbling brook. Imagine the soothing sound of the water flowing over smooth stones. Allow the sound to wash over you, calming your mind and inviting a sense of serenity.

[Pause]

Continuing your journey, you come across a peaceful clearing bathed in dappled sunlight. Feel the warmth on your skin as you step into the clearing. In the center, there's a comfortable spot to rest. As you settle in, you realize you are surrounded by gentle woodland creatures, creating a harmonious atmosphere.

[Pause]

Now, let's bring awareness to different parts of your body. Visualize the trees overhead extending their branches down to gently touch your fingertips, offering a sense of connection and support.

[Pause]

Feel the energy of the forest enveloping you, nurturing and revitalizing every cell of your body. Imagine the trees acting as conduits for grounding energy, allowing you to release any tension or heaviness.

[Pause]

As we conclude our time in the forest, take a moment to express gratitude for the healing energy it provided. Feel a deep sense of relaxation as you prepare to return to your daily life.

[Pause]

Start to bring awareness back to your breath. Begin to gently move your fingers and toes, reconnecting with your physical body. When you're ready, open your eyes, bringing the tranquility of the forest retreat with you.

Thank you for joining me in this Stress Release Through Symbolism Yoga Nidra. May the peace and strength of the forest accompany you as you move through your day. Namaste.

12. Timeless Space Journey

Welcome, dear friends. Today, we embark on a timeless space journey, where we will experience deep relaxation and detachment from the concept of time. Find a comfortable position lying down, close your eyes, and take a few moments to settle into the stillness. Inhale deeply, and as you exhale, release any tension or worries you may be carrying. Feel the support beneath you, allowing your body to melt into the ground.

[Pause]

Now, let go of all thoughts of past and future. Allow yourself to be fully present in this moment, right here, right now. Feel the sensation of your breath as it flows in and out of your body, anchoring you in the present moment.

[Pause]

Imagine yourself floating in a vast, open space, surrounded by an infinite expanse of stars. There is no up or down, no beginning or end. You are weightless, suspended in this timeless void.

[Pause]

As you float in this space, let go of any sense of time. There is no need to worry about what has happened in the past or what may happen in the future. All that matters is the present moment, where you are free to simply be.

[Pause]

Feel the peace and serenity that comes from letting go of the constraints of time. Allow yourself to sink deeper and deeper into relaxation, knowing that you are safe and supported in this timeless space.

[Pause]

Now, let's take a journey through the cosmos. Picture yourself soaring through the stars, gliding effortlessly through the universe. Feel the gentle pull of gravity as you navigate through galaxies and nebulae.

[Pause]

As you journey through space, notice how small and insignificant your problems and worries seem in the grand scheme of the universe. Feel a sense of awe and wonder at the vastness and beauty of creation.

[Pause]

Now, let's pause for a moment and simply be. Allow yourself to bask in the stillness and silence of this timeless space. Feel a deep sense of peace and contentment wash over you, knowing that in this moment, all is well.

[Pause]

As we begin to return from our timeless space journey, take a moment to express gratitude for the opportunity to experience deep relaxation and detachment from time. Know that you can return to this space whenever you need to find peace and serenity.

[Pause]

Start to bring awareness back to your breath. Begin to gently move your fingers and toes, reconnecting with your physical body. When you're ready, open your eyes, carrying the tranquility of the timeless space journey with you.

Thank you for joining me in this Timeless Space Journey Yoga Nidra. May the peace and serenity of this experience stay with you as you move through your day. Namaste.

13. Emotional Healing

Welcome, dear friends. Today, we embark on a journey of emotional healing, addressing our emotional well-being by exploring and releasing stored emotions in a safe and supportive way. Find a comfortable position lying down, close your eyes, and take a few moments to settle into the stillness. Inhale deeply, and as you exhale, release any tension or worries you may be carrying. Feel the support beneath you, allowing your body to melt into the ground.

[Pause]

Take a moment to check in with yourself emotionally. Notice any feelings or sensations that arise within you. Allow yourself to acknowledge whatever emotions may be present, without judgment or resistance.

[Pause]

Now, imagine yourself surrounded by a warm, golden light, radiating from the center of your being. This light represents love, compassion, and healing energy, offering you a safe and nurturing space to explore your emotions.

[Pause]

As you sit in this space of love and light, allow yourself to connect with any emotions that are present for you. Perhaps you feel sadness, anger, fear, or joy. Whatever you're feeling, know that it's okay to feel it. Emotions are a natural part of the human experience.

[Pause]

Now, visualize each emotion as a colorful orb of light, floating gently in front of you. Take a moment to observe the size, shape, and color of each orb. Notice how some emotions may feel heavy or dense, while others may feel light and airy.

[Pause]

With each inhale, invite these orbs of emotion to come closer to you. Allow yourself to fully embrace and experience each emotion, without trying to push it away or hold onto it. With each exhale, imagine releasing these emotions back out into the universe, allowing them to dissipate and dissolve.

[Pause]

As you continue to breathe deeply, feel a sense of lightness and freedom washing over you. Know that by acknowledging and releasing your emotions, you are creating space for healing and transformation to occur.

[Pause]

Now, let's take a moment to offer ourselves compassion and forgiveness. Repeat the following affirmations silently to yourself: "I forgive myself for any pain I've caused myself or others. I release any guilt or shame I've been carrying. I am worthy of love and acceptance just as I am."

[Pause]

Feel the weight of these affirmations lifting from your shoulders, leaving you feeling lighter and more at peace. Allow yourself to bask in the healing energy of self-compassion and forgiveness.

[Pause]

As we begin to conclude our emotional healing practice, take a moment to express gratitude for the opportunity to explore and release your emotions in a safe and supportive way. Know that you can return to this practice whenever you need to nurture your emotional well-being.

[Pause]

Start to bring awareness back to your breath. Begin to gently move your fingers and toes, reconnecting with your physical body. When you're ready, open your eyes, carrying the peace and healing of this practice with you.

Thank you for joining me in this Emotional Healing Yoga Nidra. May you continue to nurture your emotional well-being with love, compassion, and kindness. Namaste.

14. Connection with Earth

Welcome, dear friends. Today, we embark on a journey to foster a deep connection with the Earth, grounding ourselves in its energy and drawing strength from its nurturing presence. Find a comfortable position lying down, close your eyes, and take a few moments to settle into the stillness. Inhale deeply, and as you exhale, release any tension or worries you may be carrying. Feel the support beneath you, allowing your body to melt into the ground.

[Pause]

Imagine yourself lying on the soft, fertile soil of a vast meadow. Feel the earth beneath you, solid and supportive. Visualize roots extending from the soles of your feet, anchoring you deep into the earth's core.

[Pause]

As you connect with the earth beneath you, become aware of the gentle rhythm of your breath. Inhale deeply, drawing in the earth's energy through the roots of your being. Exhale fully, releasing any tension or negativity back into the earth to be transmuted and transformed.

[Pause]

Now, let's deepen our connection with the earth. Visualize a golden light emanating from the core of the earth, rising up through the layers of soil and rock. With each inhale, feel this healing energy flowing up through your roots, filling you with strength and vitality.

[Pause]

As you continue to breathe deeply, feel the earth's energy enveloping you in a warm, protective embrace. Allow yourself to surrender to this nurturing energy, knowing that you are supported and held by the earth's loving presence.

[Pause]

Now, let's take a moment to express gratitude for the earth and all its gifts. Visualize yourself surrounded by the beauty and abundance of nature, feeling a deep sense of reverence and appreciation for the interconnected web of life.

[Pause]

With each breath, feel your connection with the earth growing stronger and more vibrant. Sense the wisdom and resilience of the natural world flowing through you, empowering you to face life's challenges with grace and courage.

[Pause]

As you continue to bask in the grounding energy of the earth, allow yourself to sink even deeper into relaxation. Feel the earth's energy supporting and nourishing you on every level – body, mind, and spirit.

[Pause]

As we begin to conclude our connection with the earth, take a moment to offer a silent prayer or affirmation of gratitude. Thank the earth for its constant support and nourishment, and pledge to honor and protect this sacred bond.

[Pause]

Start to bring awareness back to your breath. Begin to gently move your fingers and toes, reconnecting with your physical body. When you're ready, open your eyes, carrying the grounding energy of the earth with you.

Thank you for joining me in this extended Connection with Earth Yoga Nidra. May you continue to cultivate a deep sense of connection and gratitude for the earth's abundant blessings. May you walk in harmony with the rhythms of nature, knowing that you are always held and supported. Namaste.

15. Candle Flame Concentration

Welcome, dear friends. Today, we will embark on a journey of concentration and focus using the image of a candle flame. Find a comfortable position lying down, close your eyes, and take a few moments to settle into the stillness. Inhale deeply, and as you exhale, release any tension or worries you may be carrying. Feel the support beneath you, allowing your body to melt into the ground.

[Pause]

Now, visualize a candle flame glowing brightly in the darkness before you. See its flickering light, dancing gracefully in the air. Notice how the flame casts a warm, golden glow, filling the space around you with its radiance.

[Pause]

As you gaze at the candle flame, feel your mind beginning to settle and focus. Allow your attention to be drawn to the gentle movement of the flame, mesmerizing you with its rhythmic dance. Notice how the flame appears to flicker and sway, yet remains steadfast and unwavering at its core.

[Pause]

Now, let's deepen our concentration on the candle flame. As you continue to gaze at its luminous glow, allow yourself to become fully absorbed in the present moment. Let go of any distractions or thoughts that arise, allowing them to fade away like wisps of smoke.

[Pause]

With each breath, feel your concentration growing stronger and more focused. Notice how the candle flame becomes the center of your awareness, drawing you deeper into a state of inner stillness and tranquility.

[Pause]

As you continue to gaze at the candle flame, feel a sense of clarity and peace washing over you. Allow yourself to sink even deeper into this state of focused awareness, knowing that you are fully present and grounded in the here and now.

[Pause]

Feel the warmth of the candle flame enveloping you like a comforting embrace, soothing your mind and calming your thoughts. Allow yourself to surrender to the gentle rhythm of the flame, allowing it to guide you into a state of deep relaxation.

[Pause]

Now, let's take a moment to express gratitude for the gift of concentration and focus. Thank the candle flame for guiding you into this state of mindfulness and presence. Feel a deep sense of appreciation for the stillness and clarity it has brought to your mind.

[Pause]

As we begin to conclude our candle flame concentration practice, take a moment to offer a silent prayer or affirmation of gratitude. Thank yourself for showing up and dedicating this time to cultivate inner peace and focus.

[Pause]

Start to bring awareness back to your breath. Begin to gently move your fingers and toes, reconnecting with your physical body. When you're ready, open your eyes, carrying the clarity and focus of the candle flame with you.

Thank you for joining me in this extended Candle Flame Concentration Yoga Nidra. May you continue to cultivate inner stillness and focus in your daily life. May the light of mindfulness guide you on your journey of self-discovery and awakening. Namaste.

16. Muscle Relaxation Journey

Welcome, dear friends. Today, we embark on a muscle relaxation journey, where we will systematically relax and release tension from each muscle group in the body. Find a comfortable position lying down, close your eyes, and take a few moments to settle into the stillness. Inhale deeply, and as you exhale, release any tension or worries you may be carrying. Feel the support beneath you, allowing your body to melt into the ground.

[Pause]

Let's begin by bringing our awareness to our feet. Take a deep breath in, and as you exhale, allow your feet to relax completely. Feel the tension melting away from your toes, the arches of your feet, and your heels. Notice the sensation of relaxation spreading throughout your entire foot.

[Pause]

Now, let's move our attention to our lower legs. Inhale deeply, and as you exhale, release any tension from your calves and shins. Feel the muscles becoming loose and limp, as if they're melting into the ground beneath you.

[Pause]

Continue to breathe deeply as we bring our awareness to our knees. With each exhale, allow your knees to soften and relax. Feel any tightness or discomfort melting away, leaving your knees feeling light and free.

[Pause]

Now, let's focus on our thighs. Inhale deeply, and as you exhale, release any tension from your thigh muscles. Feel them becoming heavy and relaxed, sinking deeper into the ground with each breath.

[Pause]

Moving up to our hips and pelvis now. Take a deep breath in, and as you exhale, allow your hips to release any tension they may be holding onto. Feel the muscles around your pelvis becoming soft and supple, as if they're gently cradling you.

[Pause]

Now, let's bring our attention to our lower back. Inhale deeply, and as you exhale, imagine any tightness or discomfort in your lower back melting away. Feel the muscles in this area becoming loose and relaxed, allowing your spine to settle into its natural alignment.

[Pause]

Continue to breathe deeply as we move up to our upper back and chest. With each exhale, allow your upper back and chest to soften and release any tension they may be holding onto. Feel a sense of openness and expansion in your chest, allowing your breath to flow freely.

[Pause]

Now, let's focus on our shoulders. Take a deep breath in, and as you exhale, allow your shoulders to drop away from your ears, releasing any tension they may be carrying. Feel the weight of your shoulders sinking into the ground, as if they're being gently supported by the earth beneath you.

[Pause]

Moving down to our arms now. With each exhale, allow your arms to become heavy and relaxed, as if they're sinking deeper into the ground. Feel any tension melting away from your upper arms, elbows, forearms, wrists, and hands.

[Pause]

Now, let's bring our attention to our neck. Inhale deeply, and as you exhale, allow your neck to lengthen and relax. Feel the muscles in your neck softening and releasing any tightness or stiffness.

[Pause]

Finally, let's focus on our face and head. With each exhale, allow your facial muscles to relax completely. Feel any tension melting away from your forehead, eyebrows, eyes, cheeks, nose, mouth, and jaw. Allow your entire face to become smooth and serene.

[Pause]

Now, take a few moments to enjoy the sensation of relaxation that permeates your entire body. Feel a sense of peace and contentment washing over you, as you surrender to the stillness and tranquility within.

[Pause]

As we begin to conclude our muscle relaxation journey, take a moment to express gratitude for the opportunity to release tension and find deep relaxation. Know that you can return to this practice whenever you need to unwind and let go.

[Pause]

Start to bring awareness back to your breath. Begin to gently move your fingers and toes, reconnecting with your physical body. When you're ready, open your eyes, carrying the sense of relaxation and ease with you.

Thank you for joining me in this extended Muscle Relaxation Journey Yoga Nidra. May you continue to cultivate relaxation and well-being in your body, mind, and spirit. May your muscles remain loose and tension-free as you move through your day. Namaste.

17. Mindful Eating Experience

Welcome, dear friends. Today, we will embark on a mindful eating experience, incorporating mindfulness into our practice by guiding you through a visualization of savoring each bite with awareness and appreciation. Find a comfortable position lying down, close your eyes, and take a few moments to settle into the stillness. Inhale deeply, and as you exhale, release any tension or worries you may be carrying. Feel the support beneath you, allowing your body to melt into the ground.

[Pause]

Imagine yourself sitting at a table in a peaceful and serene setting, surrounded by nature. Before you, there is a beautifully arranged meal, filled with colors, textures, and aromas that delight the senses. Take a moment to observe the food before you, noticing its vibrant colors and inviting presentation.

[Pause]

Now, let's begin our mindful eating experience. Start by taking a few deep breaths to center yourself and bring your attention fully to the present moment. With each inhale, feel yourself becoming more grounded and present. With each exhale, let go of any distractions or thoughts that may be pulling you away from this experience.

[Pause]

As you pick up your utensil or use your hands to take the first bite, bring your awareness to the sensation of touch. Notice the texture of the food as you hold it in your hands or bring it to your mouth. Feel its weight and temperature against your skin, allowing yourself to fully experience the tactile sensations.

[Pause]

Now, bring the food to your lips and take a small bite. Notice the flavor exploding on your taste buds as you chew slowly and mindfully. Allow yourself to savor each flavor and texture, paying attention to how the food feels in your mouth.

[Pause]

As you continue to eat, bring your awareness to the act of chewing. Notice the movement of your jaw and the muscles in your mouth as you break down the food into smaller pieces. Feel the rhythm of your chewing, allowing yourself to fully experience the process of eating.

[Pause]

With each bite, bring your attention to the sensations in your body. Notice any feelings of hunger or fullness, as well as any subtle changes in your energy levels or mood. Allow yourself to be fully present with the experience of nourishing your body with each bite.

[Pause]

As you near the end of your meal, take a moment to express gratitude for the food before you. Reflect on the journey that brought this food to your table, from the seeds planted in the earth to the hands that harvested and prepared it. Offer a silent prayer or affirmation of gratitude for the nourishment it provides.

[Pause]

As we begin to conclude our mindful eating experience, take a moment to reflect on how you feel. Notice any changes in your body, mind, or spirit as a result of this practice. Know that you can return to this experience whenever you need to cultivate mindfulness and presence in your eating habits.

[Pause]

Start to bring awareness back to your breath. Begin to gently move your fingers and toes, reconnecting with your physical body. When you're ready, open your eyes, carrying the mindfulness and gratitude of this experience with you.

Thank you for joining me in this Mindful Eating Experience Yoga Nidra. May you continue to nourish your body, mind, and spirit with awareness and appreciation in all areas of your life. Namaste.

18. Dream Exploration

Welcome, dear friends. Today, we embark on a journey of dream exploration, delving into the mysterious realm of our subconscious minds to unlock insights and creativity. Find a comfortable position lying down, close your eyes, and take a few moments to settle into the stillness. Inhale deeply, and as you exhale, release any tension or worries you may be carrying. Feel the support beneath you, allowing your body to melt into the ground.

[Pause]

As you drift into a state of relaxation, envision yourself standing at the threshold of a vast and enchanting dream world. Before you lies a swirling mist, veiling the mysteries that await beyond. Feel the anticipation and curiosity bubbling within you as you prepare to step into the unknown.

[Pause]

Now, let's begin our exploration of dreams. Take a few deep breaths to center yourself and bring your attention fully to the present moment. With each inhale, feel yourself becoming more grounded and present. With each exhale, let go of any distractions or thoughts that may be pulling you away from this experience.

[Pause]

Imagine a staircase materializing before you, its steps illuminated by a soft, ethereal light. This staircase is your gateway to the dream world, inviting you to descend into the depths of your subconscious mind. With each step you take, feel yourself sinking further into relaxation, allowing your mind to become more open and receptive to the messages and insights that await you.

[Pause]

As you reach the bottom of the staircase, find yourself standing in a lush and vibrant dreamscape, surrounded by endless possibilities. The air is alive with the hum of magic, and the landscape shimmers with an otherworldly beauty. Take a moment to marvel at the sights and sounds that envelop you, feeling the warmth of the dream world embracing you like a comforting embrace.

[Pause]

Begin to explore this dreamscape with a sense of curiosity and wonder. Allow your gaze to roam freely, taking in the intricate details of your surroundings. Notice the colors, shapes, and textures that dance before your eyes, each one holding a story or symbol waiting to be discovered. Trust in the wisdom of your inner self to guide you as you navigate this landscape of dreams and fantasies.

[Pause]

As you journey deeper into the dream world, be open to receiving insights and revelations from your subconscious mind. Pay attention to any symbols, images, or messages that may arise, trusting in the wisdom of your inner self to guide you on this journey of exploration and discovery.

[Pause]

Notice any symbols or images that catch your attention as you wander through the dream world. Pay close attention to how they make you feel and what messages they may be trying to convey. Trust in your intuition to interpret these symbols and uncover their deeper meanings.

[Pause]

As you continue to explore, allow yourself to surrender to the flow of the dream, knowing that you are safe and protected in this realm of your own creation. Embrace each moment with a sense of openness and acceptance, allowing yourself to fully immerse in the experience.

[Pause]

Now, let's take a moment to reflect on the insights and revelations that have emerged during our dream exploration. Notice how they resonate with you on a deep and profound level, offering guidance and clarity in your waking life. Trust in the wisdom of your dreams to illuminate your path and awaken your inner creativity.

[Pause]

As we begin to conclude our dream exploration, take a moment to express gratitude for the journey we have shared together. Know that you can return to this dreamscape whenever you need to reconnect with your inner wisdom and creativity.

[Pause]

Start to bring awareness back to your breath. Begin to gently move your fingers and toes, reconnecting with your physical body. When you're ready, open your eyes, carrying the insights and inspiration of your dream exploration with you.

Thank you for joining me in this Dream Exploration Yoga Nidra. May you continue to embrace the magic and mystery of your dreams, allowing them to illuminate your path and awaken your inner creativity. Namaste.

19. Colourful Energy Flow

Welcome, dear friends. Today, we will embark on a journey of colorful energy flow, guiding you to visualize and feel the vibrant stream of positive energy coursing through your body. Find a comfortable position lying down, close your eyes, and take a few moments to settle into the stillness. Inhale deeply, and as you exhale, release any tension or worries you may be carrying. Feel the support beneath you, allowing your body to melt into the ground.

[Pause]

As you enter a state of relaxation, envision a radiant ball of light hovering above you, shimmering with an array of vibrant colors. This ball of light is the source of all positive energy, waiting to infuse your being with its healing and rejuvenating power. Feel a sense of anticipation and excitement as you prepare to receive this energy into your body.

[Pause]

Now, let's begin our journey of colorful energy flow. Take a few deep breaths to center yourself and bring your attention fully to the present moment. With each inhale, feel yourself becoming more open and receptive to the flow of energy. With each exhale, let go of any resistance or blockages that may be hindering the flow.

[Pause]

Imagine the ball of light descending from above, hovering just above the crown of your head. As it draws closer, feel a gentle warmth spreading throughout your body, signaling the beginning of the energy infusion. Notice the colors swirling and dancing within the ball of light, each one representing a different aspect of positive energy.

[Pause]

Now, visualize the ball of light gently entering the crown of your head, filling you with its radiant energy. Feel the warmth spreading throughout your head, soothing and revitalizing every cell. Notice how each color of the rainbow brings its own unique qualities – red for strength and vitality, orange for creativity and passion, yellow for joy and optimism, green for healing and balance, blue for calmness and communication, indigo for intuition and insight, and violet for spiritual connection and transformation.

[Pause]

As the ball of light continues to descend through your body, feel the energy flowing freely and effortlessly. Visualize it moving down through your neck and throat, filling you with clarity and self-expression. Sense it flowing into your chest and heart, opening you to love and compassion. Feel it moving down through your abdomen and solar plexus, empowering you with confidence and personal power.

[Pause]

Now, feel the energy flowing into your hips and pelvis, grounding you and connecting you to the earth. Sense it moving down through your legs and knees, strengthening and supporting you. Feel it flowing into your feet and toes, anchoring you firmly to the ground.

[Pause]

Take a moment to bask in the sensation of vibrant energy flowing freely throughout your entire body. Notice how it uplifts and energizes you, filling you with a sense of vitality and well-being. Allow yourself to fully embrace the beauty and power of this colorful energy flow.

[Pause]

As we begin to conclude our journey of colorful energy flow, take a moment to express gratitude for the abundance of positive energy that surrounds you. Know that you can return to this visualization whenever you need to replenish your energy and uplift your spirit.

[Pause]

Start to bring awareness back to your breath. Begin to gently move your fingers and toes, reconnecting with your physical body. When you're ready, open your eyes, carrying the vibrant energy of this visualization with you.

Thank you for joining me in this Colorful Energy Flow Yoga Nidra. May you continue to embrace the beauty and power of positive energy in all aspects of your life. Namaste.

20. Breathing with the Elements

Welcome, dear friends. Today, we will embark on a journey of breathing with the elements, connecting breathwork with the natural elements of earth, air, water, and fire to create a harmonious experience with nature. Find a comfortable position lying down, close your eyes, and take a few moments to settle into the stillness. Inhale deeply, and as you exhale, release any tension or worries you may be carrying. Feel the support beneath you, allowing your body to melt into the ground.

[Pause]

As you enter a state of relaxation, envision yourself surrounded by the four elements of nature – earth, air, water, and fire. Feel their presence all around you, enveloping you in their comforting embrace. Take a moment to connect with each element, sensing their unique qualities and energies.

[Pause]

Now, let's begin our journey of breathing with the elements. Take a few deep breaths to center yourself and bring your attention fully to the present moment. With each inhale, feel yourself becoming more open and receptive to the energies of the elements. With each exhale, let go of any resistance or tension, allowing yourself to fully surrender to the experience.

[Pause]

Begin by connecting with the element of earth. Visualize yourself standing barefoot on soft, fertile soil, feeling the solid ground beneath your feet. As you inhale, imagine drawing in the stability and grounding energy of the earth. Feel it filling your body with a sense of strength and security, anchoring you firmly to the present moment.

[Pause]

Now, shift your awareness to the element of air. Feel the gentle breeze brushing against your skin, carrying with it the freshness and clarity of the air element. As you inhale, imagine breathing in the cool, crisp air, filling your lungs with vitality and inspiration. Feel it invigorating your body and mind, clearing away any stagnant energy or thoughts.

[Pause]

Next, connect with the element of water. Visualize yourself standing beside a tranquil body of water – a flowing river, a peaceful lake, or a gentle stream. As you inhale, imagine drawing in the fluidity and adaptability of the water element. Feel it flowing through your body like a gentle stream, washing away any tension or resistance. Allow yourself to surrender to the fluidity of the water, embracing its soothing and healing qualities.

[Pause]

Finally, connect with the element of fire. Visualize yourself sitting beside a warm and crackling fire, feeling its radiant warmth enveloping you. As you inhale, imagine drawing in the fiery energy of the flames, filling your body with passion and vitality. Feel it igniting the spark of creativity within you, fueling your inner fire and driving you towards your goals and aspirations.

[Pause]

Now, let's integrate all four elements into our breathwork practice. With each inhale, imagine drawing in the qualities of earth, air, water, and fire, allowing them to blend and harmonize within you. Feel their energies mingling and intertwining, creating a symphony of balance and harmony within your being.

[Pause]

As you continue to breathe with the elements, feel yourself becoming one with the natural world around you. Sense the interconnectedness of all living beings and the elemental forces that sustain life on our planet. Allow yourself to fully embrace the beauty and power of nature, knowing that you are an integral part of this wondrous tapestry of existence.

[Pause]

As we begin to conclude our journey of breathing with the elements, take a moment to express gratitude for the gifts of earth, air, water, and fire. Know that you can return to this practice whenever you need to reconnect with the elemental forces that nourish and sustain you.

[Pause]

Start to bring awareness back to your breath. Begin to gently move your fingers and toes, reconnecting with your physical body. When you're ready, open your eyes, carrying the harmonious energy of the elements with you.

Thank you for joining me in this Breathing with the Elements Yoga Nidra. May you continue to cultivate a deep connection with nature and the elemental forces that surround you. Namaste.